Pandemia as a Revision:

All you Need to Know About Symbiotic Cooperation of Microbes and a Human

Bolat Abilov

Table of Contents

About the Author

Bolat Abilov

Project Management Consultant. Fulfilled oil and gas turnkey projects with total amount increasing $5 billion and devoted 9 years to the biology investigations.

Acknowledgements

I express sincere thanks to Saule, my sister, who unconditionally supported me in all my initiatives, Lyazzat Taimanova, my groupmate, who considered them interesting, Yerkin Duiseyev, my classmate, who showed me the opportunity to express my thoughts to the world through the worldwide platform, YerzhanToyshibekov, Professor of Biology and a childhood friend, who inspired my investigations by his professionality and openness, some of their names are mentioned in the reference, and of course my sun Kaissar and my beloved woman who provided the most powerful motivation.

Introduction

Symposium of Neuro Sciences Associations that gather almost all investigators of brain activity in the world – is the most challenging intellectual events that we can only imagine.

Firstly, about 28 thousand scientists are gathered in a crowded conference hall. After some time, it seems to be an utter madness. In any restaurants, lifts or toilets, everyone around you is arguing about long neurons throughout the week. Secondly, it is a new scientific information. There are 14 thousand lectures and posters in the program, but you will be not able to see of those because of the inspired crowd of people around it. Some of these posters will be in the language that you may not know. In addition, there will be a poster that will have the results of all experiments you'll make throughout the next five years.

Besides all this, there is a common understanding that, though we are working untiringly in this field, we do not fully understand how the brain works.

Personally, I hit rock bottom after I had exhausted all possible information and feigned a general feeling of ignorance. There I was – sitting on the stairsteps of the conference hall, staring into a muddy puddle. It was then that I realized that a tiny microbe pottering in this paddle knows about the brain more than all neurobiologists together. Such a desperate conclusion has produced a recent distinguished article, "How some Microbes can Control the Brain of their Owner."

We know that primitive bacteria and viruses can use bodies of animals for their purposes in a very devious way. In order to procreate they occupy our organelles, energy, brain and change the life style... (c)[1].

It is not a figure of speech. Not a literary hyperbole for my thoughts boasting about. Rather, it is a practical result of investigations of parasites behavior.

Reading six-year-old investigations, a small amount of people believed that all epidemics were defeated in the Middle Ages. However, the last major epidemic finished somewhere during the Second World War. Clark David, a professor of law at Willamette University, revealed amazing facts about microbes, stating that they have made us as we are now, that their contribution to the modern civilization is impressive.

We, like most other people, grow up with an idea about industrial traditions and a semi-industrial society. This is the thought that every important process had a leader, "state founder," emperor, or a military commander who won any of the battles and changed the direction of the civilization development. Then we were taught that an invisible economy hand ruled everything, and that slowly following the progress helical, it would lead people to the light. However, not everything is confined to this concept. Somethings even contradict each other! Especially when it's so unclear why it took a thousand years for empires to build roads, aqueducts, and when their organization systems fell. Their *appearance* was clear, but not how they left direct successors – despite that their civilizations had writing systems, culture and knowledge, did not suffer from meteoric stone, worldwide flood, or fierce neighbors. It is also not clear why the world was lost for a hundred, or even a thousand years, and completely forgot past achievements. We do

---

[1] Robert Sapolsky. Who are we? Genes our Body Society

not have the full knowledge about how the whole worlds died and were replaced by other civilizations.

Historian Lev Gumilyov developed the universal theory of passionarity as an unexpected activation of human populations to describe how an irresistible desire to conquer seemed possible. Though everything in his nineteen books look quite colorful, and some parts are written scrupulously with convincing details, in the works of this scientist there is the concept of "passionarity", but there are no material carriers of passionarity and the mechanisms of their work.

Attempts to reproduce important events in humanity life through super powerful computer simulators, loaded with the maximum possible accurate initial parameters, were different from the reality, except some small local events. That is, until some important parameters were not considered. As soon as microorganisms were included, the white spots of canvases became colorful. They magically fulfilled the missing parts of the world picture, introduced brightness and contrast, and provided the record with expositions and proportions.

This brings up the question: who influenced the civilizations' evolution most of all?

Well, I can tell you that after eleven hours of uninterrupted reading, I was able to learn how primary microorganisms worked with scalpel and hand trowel, which changed the Earth face together with its inhabitants. These stories, even in their compressed format, are so outstanding and multivariate that to retell them without the full content wouldn't do them justice. However, in brief, I have managed to understand is that the evolution of homo sapiens. That from at least from 3,000 BC until 21th century, powerful influence of the microbe world suffered in regards to the development of population – sometimes to the point of extinction – though, more often, this happened simultaneously. Microbes – including viruses, bacteria, sporules and fungus – sometimes served as a shield for a person or group of people. Other times, they served as mass destruction, removing the territories protected by biological invaders.

In this, we can find the beginning and fall of the civilizations. For instance: the Indus river, Egypt, Rome, and Turkish empires. The fall of religions and beliefs systems like Christianity, Islam, and many others. Even the fierce horsemen of the apocalypse. All of this data makes the important point that pandemia are those who exceeded the level of death – from ½ to ¾ of the population. That, statistical recording, on the other hand, does not reflect the quality of changes.

One situation that baffled me regarded a 1816 missioner from the old world who settled in the American tribe, Koyap. This tribe began with a population of seven thousand people. Two years of coughing and sneezing reduced the population to a mere thirty Native Americans.

For the carriers of the Golden Horde from the Azov Sea until the Semirechye, a global epidemiologic disaster was the late Middle Age period of "velikaya zamyatnya." Their population was reduced to 150 thousand and their territory was also reduced until the southern oblasts of Kazakhstan. It seems that the influence of the micro world won't reduce humanity in the future.

General information about the mechanisms of microbial exposure to humans

We know that microbes come from the geological era of the planet. They lived back in the days when the spread of oxygen was a poison ancient life forms could not tolerate. Some microbes did not switch to an oxygen diet and remained in its original form. Others adapted to new conditions, learned to extract energy from it, and created the basis for the food chain of more complex forms of organisms that arose during evolution. Having learned to extract energy from everything, microbes have rightfully become ubiquitous.

Some of their homes are inseparable from our flesh, which performs many vital functions for our body. They are distributed over the surface of the skin, but a large concentration of them accompanies the food processing system, localizing in the oral cavity, intestines, and excretory system.

Microbes help us digest food by breaking it down, processing it into a digestible substrate that absorbs through the walls of blood vessels and supplies the body with energy. They specialize in different products, and, by changing taste preferences, we change the balance of specific microorganisms, increasing the content of some and reducing others in the body. But they also manipulate our taste preferences, strengthening our taste buds and causing a predisposition to certain types of products – sometimes causing dependence on them. If, for example, you can't follow a diet to lose weight, don't blame it on poor willpower. You have to overcome the resistance of microbes that are struggling to survive. They create such lust in your receptors and a cacophony in your brain that refusing to feed them brings you real pain.

It is no coincidence that the intestines are called the second brain. Its microbes produce 90% of the hormone serotonin, thanks to the regulation through which we are able to feel different degrees of satisfaction. They also produce dopamine, which increases our motivation and encourages us to act.

Through the vagus nerve, the reaction of the brain to what is happening is transmitted to the intestines. We literally experience animal fear, because it is reflected in the stomach. Sometimes we feel butterflies fluttering in our stomach. Heartburn and stomach cramps also occur due to our brains generating the stress response.

However, the intestines also have a huge reverse effect on the brain. They produce a powerful bombardment of hormones and stimulate the latter to a certain behavior.

Cooperation between humans and microbes proceeds safely for both sides as long as there is no malfunction in the human body. For example, when external conditions change, such as the appearance of new viruses. When new interaction variables arise, the nature of the relationship changes. New viruses, such as the coronavirus known as COVID-19, present a great potential for such changes.

Viruses have RNA or DNA, but they are a non-cellular form of life that needs a cell to reproduce. Such a cell can be a bacterial cell or a cell of a complex organism. The virus enters cells and embeds in the ribosomes of "home" bacteria or directly into the ribosomes of complex organisms. Where RNA, as we know, is a tape that reads instructions from the "supreme body control" – DNA for protein expression, which is responsible for about 5% of the human gene[2]. A protein, depending on the context, can be either the building material of a cell, consisting of an infinite number of organelles, or a

---

[2] Robert Sapolsky. Molecular Genetics

hormone, an axon, a neuron, etc. That is, a protein can both build and serve as a tool for controlling the body.

Embedded in the RNA, the pathogen invades the host's body, sometimes causing convulsions, blinding or deafening the body. But, what is much more interesting, is that it can also be integrated into the DNA double helix itself (i.e. it can be registered in the "central dogma of life" and settle in the command post of the host genome, where control commands are given).

How does a microbe behave in a complex organism? Like everything else in nature - only to produce copies of itself. Sometimes this is compatible with the interests of the host organism – the case of a well-lived organism with 39 trillion[3]home microbes, and sometimes not, and this is a little predictable case. In short, changes can bring new dangers, and sometimes new opportunities.

What makes the potential of microbes dangerous? First of all, the number. There are more of them than the entire human population in 10 to the 21st degree[4]. A number that is difficult to understand intuitively. The number of units is the first sign of a good survival of the species. Quantity is a resource of repetitions of replicators ' interaction between themselves and the outside world. A large number of repetitions brings a large number of results, of which remain optimal. In the case of microbes, this is an inexhaustible resource. Such a population uses the "best practice method" to select keys to any locks, no matter how complex combinations they are encoded. This is a classic evolutionary strategy that is always excellent.

Second – their simplicity. The virus has from 3 to 1,000 genes, so a small number allows them to change easily and quickly. Their rate of

---

[3] Ron Sender
[4] Clark P. David Genes Microbes Civilization

change has a huge advantage over complex organisms, such as those with 21,000 genes. It should be noted here that in complex organisms, genes are interdependent, like values in a matrix. One gene through protein expression simultaneously affects many aspects of the body's life – this is one condition, but there is another type of condition - the trait changes "if and only if the set of genes allows it"[5]. With a small number of genes, there is a small set of conditions and a smaller number of approvals that inhibit changes.

For example, a fork can extend the handle without looking back, increase or reduce the number of teeth, straighten or bend them at the desired angle - the design of this device is primitive. But changing the length of the blades in a car engine is a task that requires changes in its entire design, which then requires coordinated changes that must pass the test in several generations.

Third – the method for implementing changes. Viruses, due to the peculiarities of their structure, are able to translate DNA in their population not only in the "ancestor-descendant" chain, but also horizontally, without waiting for division in the next generation[6].

Fourth – the disease-causing virus is never completely eradicated[7]. It changes, falls into suspended animation, and masks itself from the host's immune system. It waits an hour to start producing its own copies. The waiting period may take millions of years, not hundreds or thousands. In the human body, the onset of this hour provokes diseases, stress, and the subsequent weakening. The human body has a unique set of genes. Sometimes it determines hereditary resistance to some type of interventionists, and sometimes a predisposition to diseases.

---

[5] Robert Sapolsky. Molecular Genetics
[6] Igor Vainshtok, Constantin Severinov, Andrey Schestakov, Sergey Vialov, Svetlana Schevleva, etc. Bacteria. War of the Worlds
[7] Robert Sapolsky. Who are we? Genes our Body Society

Fifth – microbes have their own propagation strategies and their own degrees of virulence. Sometimes they are bound by the habitats in which they circulate – tropical moist forests or floods of great rivers, burning lava volcanoes or in kilometers of ice. But some live in all the ecosystems in which man lives and in man himself. They receive energy even from inorganic elements such as sulfur, and are distributed by insects, rodents, pets, and from person to person through blood, skin, or airborne droplets.

Sixth. If there are no limiting conditions, the rate of replication of microbes reaches up to 200 million copies per day, which leaves them champions among all life forms in terms of reproduction rate.

Seventh. Effect on the host organism. It can be direct or indirect[8]. Penetration of ribosomes gives microbes the ability to influence the muscle and nervous system, they can take away or give energy, disrupt the work of organs, cause a nervous TIC, blind or deafen, but the ability of microbes to directly influence the brain of the host body has also been proven[9].

---

[8] Clark P. David Genes Microbes Civilization
[9] Clark P. David Genes Microbes Civilization

An example of the effect of the microbe on the brain of the owner

A classic example of such an influence in the specialized literature is toxoplasma gondi, when the parasite's area of life consists of a sequence of changes of host organisms. The parasite lives in the cat's intestines, comes out of it along with the products of metabolism and tends to return to the intestines again, because for some reason it can only breed in this intestine. The task of gondi is to make sure that the cat's feces are eaten by the rodent. To do this, the parasite must make sure that only the rodent finds this smell attractive. Once in the body, the parasite filigree acts on some neurons in the rodent's brain so that it was not eaten by a fox or a snake, but so that it got into the cat's stomach.

Surprisingly, dozens of generations of laboratory rats, in a long chain of parents no one has ever seen cats, still have an instinctive fear of them. But, in the case of gondi, the rat finds the cat's smell not only safe, but also attractive. This deactivation of the rodent's instinct provides the parasite with a return ticket home. At the same time, the social and sexual behavior of the rat remains normal, it is also smart and discriminating. It demonstrates intelligence in tasks with mazes, finds food, demonstrates aggressive, maternal and related behavior. In short, it behaves as it should. Isn't it hard to imagine that all this —with the neurons of the mammalian brain — is done by a microscopically small protozoan that has not even reached the development to be called an organism?

Brief reference

If you ask yourself how many types of pathogenic microbes there are, you will come across a long list of them and their associated epidemics. As a rule, they are modified versions of ancient ancestors. There are too many of them for easy memorization, and they are divided into systems and subsystems that can be recognized in nuances only by narrow specialists.

This abundance of microbial species, combined with their influence on complex organisms, may be part of a good explanation for how evolution has made people different. Different not only phenotypically, but different in preferences, behavior, and attitude. It is now safe to say that microbes that directly or indirectly influenced the evolution of complex organisms bear an incomplete but significant share of responsibility for this difference. The mosaic of climatic zones and the specifics of the microorganisms living in them gave the basis to divergent ones (i.e. in some cases, completely different ways of adapting human and microbial genomes to each other).

Indirect effects of microbes on human populations

Certainly, at first glance, the ability of microbes to become addicted to alcohol for an entire population rooted in a certain area will seem "impossible." The hypothesis that the symbiotic work of genomes influenced the creation of values and a cultural platform based on the product of consumption will seem implausible. Nevertheless, the process of gene influence on complex human behavior is reliably occurring, which is given extremely hard evidence[10].

Rye from the 5th century ad occupied territories from the west of France to the Russian plain, as a basic cereal crop[11]. It grows in cold, rainy climates. In the Middle Ages, as is well known, there were widespread trials of Lucifer's minions, many of whom experienced "Anthony's Fire" – an extreme degree of mental disorders that caused muscle convulsions similar to devil dances. Sometimes the "fire" manifested itself in an unstoppable stream of blasphemy and profanity. In another, already "pious" context, the infected watched in ecstasy as the heavens open with the virgin and child. The former was forced to confess their relations with the Antichrist and sent to the stake, while the latter were considered righteous and rewarded for their sanctity as far as the local parish was able. In both cases, scientists now believe that the cause of the behavior was ergot – a microbe contained in fermented rye seeds, which can be easily infected during processing or threshing. Now these microbes are considered the culprits of hallucinations and mental disorders. However, leaving the extremes, a moderate version of them causes much less neuropsychiatric severity, but at the same time leads to dependence on the consumption of products made on this culture[12].

---

[10] Richard Dawkins. The Extended Phenotype
[11] Clark P. David Genes Microbes Civilization
[12] Clark P. David Genes Microbes Civilization

Now scientists directly blame the microbes living in the human body for alcoholism[13]. It is possible that they, like the gondi, had or still have two hosts, passing from one to the other, in order to force the intermediate host to grow the rye in which they breed. Genes can do this not directly, but indirectly[14], the most reliable way is through an addiction to rye bread, kvass, beer, but even better to a strong alcoholic drink - a product that causes euphoria.

However, rye, as the main crop in northwestern Europe, by the middle of the 14th century, began to yield its niche to wheat. It can be considered a coincidence, but since then fanaticism and vivid hallucinogenic piety began to give way to moderate religious views, and later to Protestantism and pragmatism[15]. In the regions where it continues its lifecycle, and now only in the very east of Europe, ergot remained for six long centuries a fungus in the main consumer product, and presumably managed to change the genetics of the exploited population of homo sapiens because it had enough time for such changes.

Evolution performs unexpected tricks. Rye lost its monopoly power over the behavior of the intermediate host. The very need for alcohol has become an ingrained pattern of behavior, and the symbiotic genes of microbes and a higher organism have found alternative sources of obtaining it, not necessarily being tied to rye. The genes of the alcoholic microbes have enriched their host's survival tactics. They have evolved significantly, learning to provide the body with a context conducive to copious libations. It is likely that the complex organism found benefits in drinking alcohol, for example, replacing contaminated water sources. Alcohol doping apparently helped to overcome psychological barriers and carry

---

[13] O. Shishova. Who are the alcoholics in us? Are we or are they?
[14] Richard Dawkins.The Selfish Gene
[15] Clark P. David Genes Microbes Civilization

over stress. But the key may be - getting the shortest path to a state of euphoria. In the end, its use grew so that in the literature there are cases dating back to the beginning of the 20th century, when a lump of sugar soaked in alcohol was used even to calm babies.

Having learned to recognize the state of the body's propensity to consume, through feedback signals, the microbes have adapted to bring it into the desired state, each time improving the step by step practice.

Microbial genes have an even more advanced influence, not capturing individual organisms, but exploiting entire populations[16], indirectly shaping their traditions and culture, tied to the nutrition of microbes.

Over time, slowly but thoroughly, the microbes that settled in the host's body penetrated into all important areas of his life. Alcohol has become a measure of growing up and success, part of sexual and aggressive behavior, part of collaborative strategies, and an invariable feature of human dramas. Microbes-alcoholics found themselves in all spheres of social relations of the host organism, producing replications of the context, in the spirit, of the "mysterious soul" both in "great literature" and in low-standard serials and reality shows.

It is now clear that the time of the benefits that ethanol provided to the body is drawing to a close. Increase in child and female alcoholism[17], signals that the host population is oppressed by such cooperation, and the rate of negative population growth indicates a biological disaster. So, the genome of microbes drove the genome of the hosts into a dead end, but their fusion makes it difficult to distinguish one from the other.

---

[16] Clark P. David Genes Microbes Civilization
[17] T. Vysothskaya. Alcoholism in Russia and its consequences

Coexisting concepts of survival, such as the cult of productivity and the development of technological competitiveness, are cognitively obvious, but probably should rely on other consumption, in which alcohol will take a more modest position. But for this, not only alcoholic microbes must yield their niche to other microbes, but also the gene of a complex organism linked to the trait must be neutralized. But why would they do that? Concepts that interfere with the lines of basic consumption are themselves pushed to the periphery and have little chance of survival, since this requires more than cognitive levers that cannot be applied upon waking up one Monday morning.

A humanitarian catastrophe frightens society with its inevitability. Therefore, from time to time, scientists make sensational statements that the gene for alcoholism has been discovered (once again) and even some name has been assigned to it. Together with this statement, there is an encouraging announcement of a miracle pill, but no one was able to see it in wide sale. And the point may not be a blunder of scientists, but the fact that the gene does not intend to die and mimics it much faster than researchers discover. In addition, it is linked to other genes, and neutralizing it can have far-reaching consequences.

This raises a host of questions about artificial genome editing technology. For example, such a plan: it may be better not to look for ways to destroy all the time elusive genes, but to find an opportunity to use the genes for resistance to alcoholism, which the Japanese and Chinese have[18]? Maybe these genes will cope better with the disease by speaking their own language?

So. The epicenter of the circulation of microorganisms is probably still the area corresponding to the growth conditions of rye, but

---

[18] Svetlana Borinskaya. Drunkenness Gene

having taken root in the intestine and embedded in the DNA of the host organism, the microbes found ways to survive using a wider scale and penetrating to higher levels of influence. By freeing themselves from the dependence of the maternal cereal culture, they made the host's organism resourceful both in switching to other sources of alcohol and in expanding the context of its consumption. Perfectly settled, they have no intention of leaving their habitat, and so far, they are doing it successfully.

This example shows how unpredictable the long-term influence of microorganisms on the genome and brain of the host can be.

As a result of long and complex interactions, as well as changing conditions, different groups of human populations have received different predispositions.

In some cases, the synthesis of conditions requires from both the higher and the simplest genomes coexisting in one organism, an increase in activity, productivity, a better response to changes in the environment, better learning ability, greater memory and quick wits.

Microbes, of course, do not know anything about high fashion or compound interest, they do not share any beliefs of the owner, but they know which signals they feel better, and which ones worse.

As mentioned earlier, microbes have a multi-systemic effect on higher organisms. Microbial colonies communicate in the host's body through biochemical reactions. They express the same hormones as in humans, such as norepinephrine, dopamine and serotonin, influencing human mood and behavior. In some cases, the synthesis of primordially selfish strategies is an example of a randomly formed mutual benefit.

How does this happen?

Using the same lock-and-key process, in which symbiotic genes (i.e. human genes and genes of microbes) select the most favorable modes of interaction.

If the predominant group of microbes is configured to benefit energetically from the activity of the host's brain, it will no doubt stimulate it. Of course, by forming not the thoughts themselves, but a predisposition to the active work of the brain. Not ideas, but the quality of communication in neural networks. Not clues, but better metabolism of the amygdala, cortex, and hippocampus, able to recognize, analyze and learn. Not productivity, but the highest degree of motivation.

Microbes will not plant an invention on an engineer, but they can boost the activity and performance of his brain, supplying him with blood, nutrients and hormones, helping him create mental abstractions and stimulating his rewards. Again, the advanced influence of the gene extends to the formation of a productivity context in one or even several populations with divergent modes of interaction.

The result of the pandemics of the Middle Ages was a positive selection of genes endowed with small anomalies. Perhaps the result of the European and Asian plague was the selection of people with mild obsessive-compulsive disorder, expressed in a slightly greater than usual, anxiety, pedantry and ritualism entrenched in the population due to the habit of more careful application of hygiene measures, which it could have been in their time. These "sanitary" genes could spread, and in a few centuries become a feature of the "portrait of the nation." This could happen due to the transfer of mild anxiety to all objects of life. For example, a little more attention to detail, a more persistent desire for functionality, accuracy and reliability, as well as increased scrupulousness in everything. The author has not come across studies that directly confirm these conclusions for specific populations, but indirect[19]studies reveal the advantages of very mild forms of schizotypality for their adaptation in the genome.

In conditions of natural restrictions, such as island ones, where, due to natural restrictions and high competition with neighbors, intensive rather than extensive development of advantages is especially important, it is possible to shift the emphasis to other ways of productivity.

For example, from time to time, outbreaks of brain hyperactivity can have an effect due to powerful spontaneous bursts of activity, when everything routinely current seems incredibly slow, dumb, moving at snail speeds. During such periods, more often than usual, insights and high-quality breakthroughs come. Once spread, this trait can change the entire population. However, such outbursts can be accompanied by an unbridled thirst for consumption, attacks of antisocial behavior and hypertrophied aggression. People with bipolar disorder are thought to have these symptoms[20]. Individuals have to pay for the bursts of activity with prolonged periods of melancholy and depressive states.

This disorder has a pronounced genetic factor, and on average, a low recurrence rate around the world, except that England with 4 million carriers [21] creates an unusually high cumulation. Such saturation, turned into the recent past, presupposes the concentration of active carriers of high intelligence, prone to non-

---

[19] Robert Sapolsky. Schizophrenia. Martin Moler gene upgrade. Why we are using an outdated body model in a new world model and how to fix it.
[20] BBC. Bipolar disorder
[21] BBC. Bipolar disorder

standard behavior. It seems to be sufficient to gain a critical mass to induce local and then global changes. Which, in general, was embodied by the British Empire.

Who knows if the most mysterious epidemic of the Middle Ages, the "English sweating fever" that broke out in Tudor England in 1485 and ended in 1551, which greatly thinned its population, is not responsible for this? In settlements such as Cambridge and Oxford, it took away about half of the population, but, for unclear reasons, bypassed places of concentrated residence of inhabitants of Celtic origin. Apparently, that is why it is called "English." The outbreak in Germany, Sweden and Norway probably does not refute this opinion. From some sources of the description, it follows that the disease affected the body in just a few hours, causing intense fever, without having time to leave ulcers. And as if it was possible to escape from it if you take reactive response measures, and this facilitated by quick-wittedness, enterprise and the ability of a person to act quickly and calmly. The epidemic has obviousprobably shifted the population ratio in favor of the latter.

It remains to be wondered if England would have left the bosom of the papacy, there would have been a victory over the Armada, the Bank of England would have been invented, there would have been a cascade of bourgeois, trade, financial and technological revolution without people of non-standard thinking, had they cling to the canons of the "normality" of their time. Perhaps part of this disorder should be thanked for a galaxy of geniuses of culture, science and military affairs, such as, for example, Alan Turing or the Liverpool Four became.

On the west coast of the Atlantic, there has been a new, sustained interaction between the genome of the Old World and the genome of the microbes circulating in America, and it induces subtle but accumulating differences that will undoubtedly manifest something new.

However, while giving relations to the influence of microbes on the success of some human populations, one must also remember those whom they sent to the Kingdom of the Eternal Hunt, who did not have mutually beneficial symbiotic cooperation with the microcosm, and whose chronicle was cut short.

What does COVID-19 bring?

The past history cannot predict a lot about real consequences of the certain COVID-19 virus.

There is no developed verified data about the so-called "Chinese Virus" from respected magazines, such as *Science*, as on the date of writing this report. Until present day, the nature of the COVID-19 virus is not known. But partially collected information says that this virus has a sequence of reactions. After the Wuhan immune system breaker comes excitation of bacterial pathogens. As together, with respiratory disease, the virus has a multisystem effect and influences on blood coagulability, kidneys, heart and brain.

Long lasted activity of the coronavirus forecasts influence of the virus genome on DNA of a human body.

The COVID-19 virus may act completely different on different populations. The virus interacts with the circulated microbes so much different as climatic zones – extremely continental, temperate, tropical etc. – this diversity is increased many times due to diversity of a diet, and even more due to variants of genomes of higher organisms.

What cannot be predicted?

It seems unlikely to predict theoretically exactly what changes will occur with certain populations of people.

Taking into account the widely available information that coronaviruses have RNA with unusual up to 30 thousand base pairs, this should guarantee the extraordinary potential of virus mutations when interacting with ribosomes of "domestic" bacteria, as well as ribosomes and human DNA, and, probably, this promises an active influence of the virus on a complex organism.

If I understand correctly the theory of natural automata[22], its essence lies in the fact that in each case of interaction of simple elements, such as "0" and "1," which occur according to simple local rules, different results come out. This difference is not due to the same type of input data and the influence of local conditions. In our case, the genes of the virus - the causative agent of the reaction, the genes of bacteria circulating in a specific environment and the genes of a complex organism - will interact.

The results of the first interaction of the genome of microbes and the human genome will serve as the initial data for the second iteration of the interaction. The results of the second iteration will become the input data for the third, and so on. From iteration to iteration, the divergence of results in each organism will increase.

In many of such interactions, as follows from the theory, nothing new is formed. In a very small amount, something neutral and uninteresting is formed. But in one case in a billion, and maybe less often, something dynamic and capable of radical transformations

---

[22] Stephen Wolfram

can break out. This means that after several rounds of interactions with microbes, tiny differences in the genome can cause huge differences between them.

On the other hand, following the same theory, the differences will not scatter to different ends of the universe, but are structured into several general patterns. The point may be that with a large run-up of results, there are a limited number of solutions. According to the results of selection, lines that have received advantages as a result of mutations, lines with neutral adaptation and lines of extinction can be formed.

Everyone, of course, would like to guess in advance what rules the selection will follow, but now it looks like an unpredictable process.

Forecasting requires powerful software that can handle an unimaginable amount of data; experiments with legions of table flies and laboratory animals. Of course, you need smart heads capable of processing, interpreting the results, as well as those who have the imagination and determination to make decisions, to understand the consequences of actions or inaction. Most likely, this will result in a variety of prediction models, of which only an insignificant part, covered with a heap of ethereal predictions, will be verified by reality. But having such results is still better than not having them.

Isolation

Compulsory quarantine, like any marinating people in confined spaces, even at home, has always been considered a form of punishment that has a punitive meaning. Even a partial restriction of freedom of movement has a negative imprint.

The practice of isolation, at least in the summer of 2020, when, according to the prevailing theories, the activity of the virus was supposed to go down, brought Kazakhstan to the anti-record in terms of the number of infected and deaths from coronavirus per capita. The virus, apparently, did not read theories, and forced immobility weakened the working state of the lungs, increased the vulnerability of diabetics, and the sudden deprivation of stress caused stress and a sharp deterioration in all predisposed people.

Added to this were social factors. In the summer of 2020, it was not possible to hide from the stream of toxic information about COVID-19 that poured "from every microwave." Personal messengers are tired of broadcasting a stream of obituaries and a long line of condolences. We were involved in a chain reaction - the loss of loved ones, the closure of businesses, forced layoffs, an increase in debts, a collapse in living standards and family dramas that broke out. All this against the backdrop of endless high-profile corruption scandals with the creation of artificial shortages and a black market for drugs, the helplessness of doctors and a shortage of beds in hospitals, as well as the exposure of the weakness and managerial incapacity of the authorities, which have no other than repressive responses.

This cannot be repeated.

But, on the other hand, gatherings of people, dictated by the most powerful pressure of tradition, caused a rapid increase in the number of infected. Unfortunately, the customs of holding mass celebrations, sharing a meal, hugging and kissing turned sideways to us.

Quarantine has caused a cascade of well-known changes in the economic environment, and some of them have every reason to gain a foothold for a long time.

What matters to me is that the time freed from the need to stay in transport was used to find and study things that could not reach my hands.

In general, social distancing guidelines to avoid sneezing and tactile contact with common items seems to have changed the culture of interaction.

Allies

What we can be sure of is that if the infection passes into the bacterial part, the Safari season opens on the pathogenic bacteria from the side of bacteriophages. This oldest form of life is about 3 billion years old. Phages are viruses, natural antiseptics, targeting bacteria. Clinging to them, the phages inject their DNA into the bacteria, destroying them from the inside and turning their remains into their own food, and with the disappearance of the nutrient medium, the phages themselves fall into suspended animation. Those. their reproduction is strictly proportional to the change in the number of bacteria.

This is an example of unintentional altruism that benefits both sides. The benefit of egoistic gene strategies is that bacteriophages satisfy their needs without directly harming the cells of higher organisms.

Meanwhile, bacteriophages are not universal, each is narrowly specialized for only one type of bacterium, and 42 species of phage are needed to destroy such bacteria as Staphylococcus aureus.[23]

Then there are a couple of caveats.

First, it is important to emphasize that phages do not cause "direct" harm, but they can force bacteria to inject toxic substances harmful to the human body (i.e. cause indirect harm).

Second, "do not harm" does not mean that phages see it as their mission to save a complex organism. This is the business of the organism itself.

---

[23]Uta Kroycha. Bacteriophages and their role in medicine

Antibiotics

A special word must be said about antibiotics. Howard Flory, 20th Century Nobel Laureate, said that synthetic antibiotics should be used only in matters of life and death, and spoke out against their free sale in pharmacies. This is due to a double negative effect. On one hand, the rate of growth of microbial resistance, and, on the other, with the destruction of the beneficial microflora of the body.

But the man, not fully understanding the consequences, expressed his intention to control the microcosm through the development of antibiotics, and, for some time, they allowed themselves to be considered defeated.

However, in the 1990's, the status quo changed. Antibiotics, as it turned out, kill strong bacteria, but leave weak. But weak bacteria are still capable of colonization and degeneration. The new antibiotic makes the generation of resistant microbes even more adaptable and even more aggressive. In the first decade of the 21th century, 60% of new generation microbes turned out to be insensitive to antibiotics. Now there are several strategies for combating microbes with synthetic antibiotics:

- Microbes have learned to change their appearance, which the antibiotic simply does not recognize.

- They learned to create a protective belt around themselves, through which it is impossible for the medicine to break through

- They learned to produce substances that can destroy the antibiotic when it has not yet had time to reach its goal

- Microbes have learned to feed on antibiotics, destroy them inside themselves, and even hunt them

These strategies are transmitted by microbes via RNA or DNA as instructions for leveling each type of antibiotic. Moreover, as we remember, viruses transmit them horizontally across the entire population of the range at once.

It must be remembered that, using antibiotics and vaccines, a person changes not only his microflora, he changes the biology of his immediate environment. In new circumstances, this imposes social responsibility on him. You need to ask the questions:

- What kind of synthetic hell should the vaccine carry in order to be guaranteed to destroy them?

- Will vaccinated people survive it?

- Should we use synthetic means to tease fate and open a portal to something unknown and immeasurably sinister?

Genes. Genomic slavery and technology

We all are well aware of the three-dimensional model of DNA, the 3 billionth code, encoded with a sequence of nitrogenous bases A, T, C, G, presented on the basis of the discovery made by Watson and Crick in the middle of the twentieth century.

It contains a personal history of evolutionary development from the first replicators to you. This is a chronicle of the transmission of gene copies and their typos (mutations) from generation to generation, among which most of the typos were neutral in nature, and a minority gave either advantages or flaws that manifested themselves in the context of interaction with the environment. Genes affect the phenotype, the sensitivity to irritation factors, the ability... in almost all areas of life. Genes are not a guarantor of the manifestation of a particular property, rather their influence is considered in categories of high, medium or low probability, such as the probability of winning the sprint distance or getting schizophrenia. But, in some cases, genes provide 100% predestination for the realization of a trait, such as Huntington's Disease.

Since evolution is a blind process. Random shuffling does not concern itself with the extinction or prosperity of some chosen combination of genomes in the future. Will the population adapt to new conditions or other species will occupy its niche? Evolution does not bother.

But man, having achieved success in genome sequencing, makes active attempts to introduce control into evolution, i.e. artificially, at your own discretion, influence its process. This leads to some moral collisions, but the survival motive is tempting more and more people to edit their own genome.

The editing tools in biohacker technology are laboratory viruses with an embedded genome. They, according to the already known principle, penetrate the cell and inject their DNA into it, trying to register in the host's code, but viruses do not penetrate into all types of cells.

Cheaper, burgeoning genetic technologies are growing faster than smartphone technologies. Buying a DNA strand sequence over the Internet for $ 10-20 creates a huge temptation to genetically alter oneself, even in a makeshift way. It seems that there is no power to cope with the desire of nihilists to build breasts, build muscles, eat and not get fat, eliminate or reduce the likelihood of diabetes, cancer and heart disease, etc., as well as become smarter, postpone extinction and prolong life with the help of injections and without the help of doctors.

The SCRIPR-CAS 9 Scissors technology exploded the concept of genetic therapy in 2013 by replacing bacterial gene sites in 321 sites. Then she found development on mice, and later in China on the embryos of human embryos.[24].

The original process is based on the fact that the first blade of the GRNA or Guide RNA scissors finds a given sequence of the gene code in the genome, and the second CAS 9 enzyme delivers the required genetic material to the site. The unwanted gene material is then removed and the desired version is inserted. This process is being improved and modernized very quickly. If this operation looks mechanically filigree, and the question of what to remove or what to implant is entirely the responsibility of the person concerned, it remains only to ask about safety.

---

[24] Martin Moler gene upgrade. Why we are using an outdated body model in a new world model and how to fix it.

As mentioned earlier, tens of thousands of genes in the human genome have complex connections with each other, and the consequences of a small change in it can be analogous to the "flapping of the wings of a butterfly in Korea that provoked a hurricane in California." Some genes work only in pairs, so more than one trait changes, and some can cause a cascade of changes. Figuratively speaking, in order for a beautiful priest to grow, but at the same time, the kidneys did not fail, it may become necessary to make thousands of genome edits, and in a year, when it turns out that because of them, the aging mechanism was activated prematurely, tens of thousands more will be required to suppress it, etc. etc.

Goldman's dilemma – "Do you agree, as a result of gene therapy, to win Olympic gold in exchange for ending life in 5 years?"– metaphorically reflects the essence of retribution for an artificial imbalance.

This can be further complicated by the fact that the designer focuses on the existing external environment, without considering unpredictable changes in the future. For instance, with the pandemic of COVID-19 or its strains is such an unforeseen situation.

Currently, gene therapy methods are described in terms of "considered safe" rather than "safe." In order to declare the reliability of the technology, many years of observations are needed, tested in different conditions. In addition, often we are talking about tests on rodents, cats or dogs that have a device similar to humans. But a person is still more complicated than cats and dogs, and if, after some influence on animals, they, for example, demonstrate the same ingenuity as before the experiment, this does not say anything about harm to humans. Our ingenuity is not limited by the speed of finding a way out of the maze. The results of experiments on animals cannot be extrapolated to humans, if only because we do not have their metabolic system, our olfactory organs are not responsible for 40% of the perception of the world, and they do not have the same brain, the number of neurons and connections between them. We don't catch mice for dinner, and they didn't keep balance sheets or design chemical plants either before or after the experiment. Those. the comparison will never be correct.

Gene therapy looks very promising and not as dangerous as antibiotics, but its advanced technologies, although they are developing by leaps and bounds, are still young, and have practically no proven human experience.

Say goodbye to viruses forever?

George Church came to the idea of creating a human body completely resistant to viruses, as I understand it, its originality is based on the weak point of viruses - their inability to produce protein without using foreign cells. In the human body, a codon consisting of a combination of three nucleotide residues encodes a sequence of amino acids in the structure of a cell. The interaction occurs when the codon of the cell reads the codon of the virus and recognizes it as complementary. The cells of complex organisms have a greater variety of codons; one amino acid can be encoded in several ways. The idea is to exclude codons of the cell complementary to the codons of the virus, so that the cell simply cannot read the codon of the virus and thus exclude their interaction. That is, to minimize the functional diversity of cell codons to the scheme: one codon - one amino acid.

This will be possible only with the help of a radical rewriting of the human genome, about 400 thousand edits, i.e. a significant part of the "code of life," which is not excluded by the author himself. The idea looks exciting in its novelty, but there are a few questions worth asking:

What will be the direct and indirect implications for interactions with 39 trillion domestic bacteria?

How far will the edited people remain a link in their genetic chain and how much are the products of design? How will this affect human genetics in general?

Microbes have proven their viability, safely multiplying for 15 years in open space at the Mir Orbital Station, they were also found in the reactor of the Chernobyl Nuclear Station[25]. What happens if, as a result of mutation, viruses pick up the keys to human codons? Wouldn't a "completely resistant organism" become "completely vulnerable" to all Egyptian executions? After all, now it will be removed from the warranty period.

[25] Igor Vainshtok, Constantin Severinov, Andrey Schestakov, Sergey Vialov, Svetlana Schevleva, etc. Bacteria. War of the Worlds

What should ordinary people do before finding a panacea?

You should probably use the Japanese folk wisdom: "Solve small issues, big ones decide themselves." (c)

It seems to me that this task needs to be divided into two tightly linked parts.

First. Reduce the brutality of pathogen intervention.

Bearing in mind that, in addition to personal danger, the virus serves as a trigger for a reaction, prompting bacteria and fungi to attack a complex organism, it is necessary to reduce the concentration of the latter in places where a person is staying. This is especially true in areas in your home where mold can form (i.e. fungus).

Microbes several nanometers in size can contain up to 500 units of fungus per cubic meter of air in such places, and several dozen are enough to infect a person with a weakened immune system. These places include not only sinks, bathrooms and washing machines, which are regularly disinfected, but also air conditioners, unventilated entrances, damp walls and darkened corners with moisture, which are likely to be seeded with fungi of the aspergillus genus. Under natural conditions, these microbes live in compost heaps, but a weakened organism may well pass for it. They multiply in the lungs and travel from the lungs to the heart, brain and legs.

Not only surfaces, but also the air in these rooms must be periodically treated with an antiseptic, preventing invasion through the respiratory tract.

Naturally, when you come home, you also need to process your clothes and shoes, not to mention regular hand washing - the absolute record holders in collecting microbes.

I think, without an urgent need, people need to beware of places where antibiotics are regularly used - factories that produce new strains of microbes, such as hospitals[26].

Second. Increasing your own resistance to viruses.

First of all, I would like to remind you about the essence of the signaling system in the body numbers and the state of the environment. This information can. Microorganisms have something similar to a collective mind, they regularly communicate, throwing out biochemicals to get feedback about their inform the microbes about unfavorable conditions, give the command to stop dividing and fall into suspended animation. Or, on the contrary, to report that the Paradise for reproduction has come, and then the division of microbes becomes pathogenic.

Human cells also emit signals about their condition, which are received by both their own systems and microbes. Signals about the healthy state of the body are suppressed by pathogens, they cannot gain a quorum for the unfolding of disease-causing scenarios and humbly go into hibernation. Life-affirming signals are also drowned out by their own mortal genes, which are responsible for initiating the body's withering. This happens because the gen coalition is convinced of the viability of the organism and decided to give it a new loan. This development will be enthusiastically supported by the Legion of domestic bacteria, kindly providing an Arsenal of their best services to ensure the viability of the host.

---

[26] Dirk Bokmul. The Secret Life of Household Microbes: All About Bacteria, Fungi and Viruses

Nutrition, of course, determines your composition of bacteria in the gut, and therefore affects the brain, bacteria have you to taste preferences, behavior, and diseases. But all these factors are individual and can be considered in the context of the influence of the gene.

Nevertheless, there is a panacea, not without reason claiming to be universal, probably you have already guessed what is going to be discussed.

Modern research suggests that the lion's share of positive signals is reproduced by the moving muscle system, which I will discuss in more detail in figures and facts in the next book.

Cardio and especially strength training, the role of which is still underestimated, come to the forefront of this process. These loads mobilize the work of all body systems: the musculoskeletal system, cartilage, respiratory system, blood supply, digestion, internal organs and the brain[27]. Signals such as circulating oxygen-rich blood, fat burning, increased insulin sensitivity, supporting neurogenesis and protecting neurons from destruction, and the collapse of prolonged stress, tell the genes that the body has an unwavering intention to live.

Dozens of studies report on the amazing success of our contemporaries who took up physical therapy, and even at a respectable age managed to improve their health, rejuvenate and restore the joy of life. This effect is observed not only in increasing the body's endurance and working capacity of organs, not only in skin rejuvenation, and not only in the prevention of diabetes, cancer and cardiovascular diseases, it is manifested in increased concentration, coordination and memory improvement. For

---

[27]Shtipler. Muscles, how are you?

example, loads make us not only higher-faster-stronger, but also smarter. And, as mentioned above, the signals of healthy cells have a positive effect on resistance to infectious epidemics.

This phenomenon is based on the work of our ancient genes, which have a single goal – survival. The potential of these long-lived genes, who live thousands or even millions of years, will be discovered for many, many years to come.

Compulsory quarantine, like any marinating people in confined spaces, even at home, has always been considered a form of punishment that has a punitive meaning. Even a partial restriction of freedom of movement has a negative imprint.

Conclusion

Once more about genes

Nature itself gently control the adaptation processes.

Thus, in 1976, Sr. Richard Dawkins believed the hypothesis that genes may prolong the life up to 150 and 200 years in case of radical conditions change, but he did not consider artificial genome change. In response to his hypothesis, skeptics can reasonably refer to telomeres located at the of DNA and restricting quantity of cells division and consequently preventing from life prolongation. This dogma seems to be undisputable.

But after studying evolution of species for some time, you stop to be surprised how insignificant things lead to unbelievable changes and how easily the evolution gets free from sacramental taboo, passing them in a masterful way. Mechanism of natural mutation exists for this.

This ancient homo sapiens amphibious hidden at the seacoast from sea predators made the first difficult step to the land, perhaps he also had tribesmen – skeptics twisting a finger at a temple. How these wisemen might know the result of his absurdity.

Of course, scientists' views on possible and impossible varies faster – from one system of dominating views to another. And when one dogma fails and the next one starts, certainly good explanations will be found for it. Investigators will compete in faultless arguments disclosing this phenomenon, and incidentally they will indulgently remember about bald and narrow-minded orthodox scientists of the past who follow the attributes of their scientific greatness not accepting the wind of changes And blah-blah –blah. It is a typical story.

But the coronavirus case goes beyond the borders of ordinary consequences, not fully informed part of population may become an experimental field, thanks to or to the contrary to the modern scientific standard. I suppose that most of us do not want to derail the life plans because of the COVID-19 invasion, but also do not want to be a genetically improved version of the 2020 season.

Do scientists make mistakes? Definitely. Our history is full of such stories. Quite often changeability depends on "scientific glasses" that are in fashion at a certain period of time. Mistakes are a norm. The important thing is that mistakes of any genius man do not become a fixed idea of a super powerful billionaire decided to play messianism. As long as this symbiosis lead to fatal consequences. It is better for scientific thoughts to be victims than for people.

The essential point is not to save money on vaccines and doctors by doing natural and affordable preventive measures including efficient sanitizers, outdoor fitness equipment, a pair of trainers and several T-shirts, the real point is regularly to call for the nature automatic health-promoting patterns. With such an insistence, we increase our chances of not only overcoming the COVID-19 virus, but we may also be able to use its new possibilities. We have to send signals systematically allowing the nature to do her part of a delicate complex work on regulating complicated balances.

Best regards and see you next time!